# Table of Contents

Bladder Cancer Survival Rates in Relation to Age: A Comprehensive Analysis

# Breaking Down Bladder Cancer Survival Rates By Age

# 1. Introduction

The factors and statistics affecting the survival rate of bladder cancer are many and shifting. In this article, we're going to focus specifically on age and how it affects survival rates for NMIBC and MIBC. Of course, when most people are first diagnosed, bladder cancer survival rates can sway your perspective and give you hope or dread. A couple of comforting statistics are that over half of bladder cancer cases occur in people over 75. When survival rates compare age groups nearly a decade apart, so many other factors are at play. In this article, we hope to best serve people who want these statistics by age, no matter how nuanced they may be.

Bladder cancer survival outcomes are data that doctors, patients, and caregivers heavily rely on when discussing this type of cancer. Further broken down, these data are generally based on factors like gender, severity, stage, location, and so on. In this article, we're going to tackle one survival rate, and that's how age affects bladder cancer survival rates. We're going to explore the specific survival rates for non-muscle invasive bladder cancer (NMIBC) and muscle invasive bladder cancer (MIBC) in relation to age.

# 2. Understanding Bladder Cancer

# 2.1. Definition and Types

# 2.2. Epidemiology and Risk Factors

# 3. Survival Rates in Bladder Cancer

Five-year relative survival for bladder cancer among all individuals who were diagnosed in 2008-2014 was 77.7 percent. Bladder cancer has a modest five-year relative survival rate. As the patient ages, the age-related survival price rises. Two-thirds of individuals with bladder cancer are over the age of 65, and the median age at diagnosis is 73. Survival rates by bladder cancer grade or stage are also collected by the Surveillance, Epidemiology, and End Results (SEER) program of the National Cancer Institute. This data provides the number of individuals with a specific type of bladder cancer who have lived for a certain amount of time after being diagnosed. Although grouped survival statistics do not provide individualized survival estimates, they assist people better comprehend how much current bladder cancer recurrence rates can affect survival among those with bladder cancer of the same type and stage.

The survival rate for bladder cancer reflects the number of individuals who live after being diagnosed with the disease. Five-year net survival rates for bladder cancer vary because they reflect the different tracks taken by the patients and, to a smaller degree, the duration of follow-up. The factors that have a significant impact on the overall survival rates are tumor extent, severity of the tumor (including tumor category and tumor stage), patient age, and general health. Other survival statistics for bladder cancer include five-year relative survival by race, including

1987-2012 and 2008-2014. Five-year relative survival is stratified by stage and age. Local and regional disease is associated with a higher five-year relative survival rate than metastatic or unknown disease, whereas higher five-year relative survival rates correlate with earlier age at diagnosis.

## 3.1. Factors Affecting Survival Rates

Impact of age on bladder cancer: Age continues to be a factor that influences a patient's survival rate. When considering the form of cancer in the US, survival rates are separated into one of two age brackets. The first is broken down into 0-29 years old. The range grows in 10-year increments to a final range split for 80+ years of age. While bladder cancer is more common among older individuals, there are still plenty of young and middle-aged patients. If we look at the overall total of the range split, the life expected survival rate of all races is about 77.3 for males and 79.3 for females.

Factors that may have an impact on survival rates include the patient's age, overall health, the stage of the cancer, the grade of the tumor, timely treatment, and the patient's response to treatment. Bladder cancer, like all forms of cancer, is varied and carries different prognoses. For instance, a diagnosis of non-muscle invasive cancer in stage 0 has a 5-year survival rate of approximately 89%. A diagnosis of a muscle-invasive cancer in stage 3, on the other hand, sees a 5-year survival rate of only 47.3%. In addition to stage, survival rates can change when considering other factors such as grade. For stage 0 cancers, high-grade tumors have a lower probability of survival than low-grade tumors. This is unfortunate when coupled with the fact that high-grade tumors are more common in unhealthy individuals and older patients.

## 3.2. Overall Survival Rates

It is worth noting that the survival rate of bladder cancer refers to the overall effectiveness of treatment for the entire population of individuals with this type of cancer. Bladder cancer is staged on a scale from 0 to 4 to assess the severity and spread of the cancer. The TNM system, used by the University of Chicago in 2017, is used to determine the stage of the cancer. These statistics are based on data collected over a period of 5 years by the National Cancer Institute. The numbers provided are for cases without continuous chemotherapy. On average, about 77 out of 100 people are still alive one year after their cancer is diagnosed. Over a period of 5 years, this number drops to about 70 out of 100. Patients who are 65 years old or older may have a slightly lower survival rate compared to younger patients with bladder cancer. Some individuals with bladder cancer have more aggressive forms of the disease and, if the condition does not improve, have a worse prognosis.

Overall survival rates: Around 77% of people survive bladder cancer, making it past the first year. 70% of people will survive at least another 5 years, making the 5-year survival rate. Without further treatments, people with the most advanced stages of bladder cancer are unlikely to survive 20 years or more. However, if the cancer is removed from the body and does not return for 5 years, it is less likely to come back, although there is no guarantee.

# 4. Age as a Key Factor

# 4.1. Impact of Age on Survival

# 4.2. Age-Specific Survival Rates

# 5. Research Methods

# 5.1. Data Sources and Study Design

# 5.2. Statistical Analysis Techniques

# 6. Findings and Interpretations

The Kaplan-Meier method was used to calculate each actuarial survival point, and the log-rank test was used to evaluate survival differences among the four age and gender groups. The relationships between the factors and CSS were further identified with the Cox proportional hazard models. The Akaike information criteria (AIC) and Bayesian information criterion (BIC) indices, along with likelihood ratio tests, might demonstrate variations in model fit and effectiveness. In summary, this study provided a comprehensive overview of the prognosis of age- and sex-stratified bladder cancer patients, as well as potentially viable therapeutic interventions in older and female bladder cancer patients.

This study has systematically investigated the differences in bladder cancer-specific survival rates between age groups. It used age-stratified bladder cancer patients from the Surveillance, Epidemiology, and End Results database and the Kaplan-Meier method. Cox proportional hazard models and the AIC/BIC indices were applied to evaluate the associations. It found that the survival of bladder cancer worsens with increasing age, though the impact of sex on survival decreased with increasing age. Positive lymph node status has a large effect on reducing survival in all age and sex groups. This study shows that older patients and female patients have a worse prognosis when diagnosed with bladder cancer. It is critical to effectively manage the indicators and employ more aggressive therapeutic strategies in older and female patients with BC in the future.

Further, middle-aged seniors (73 to 78) can expect a roughly 97 percent 1-year relative survival rate with a low about 2 percent risk of death in the 1-year post-diagnosis (i.e., (1 minus 97) = 0.03 (or 3%)). Compared to median survival by age group - with a median survival of 1.85 years of seniors aged 96 and 2.91 years of seniors aggregated but excluding those 89 and 90 but re-aggregated to follow the main report's age categories. In this section of the report, we present the detailed determinations by age. To be clear, the age figures cut off at that year minus 1 (e.g., adults 47 are analyzed in the age range 45-49 years) and are thus of the adult population who turn that age in the year of diagnosis. Overall, as the main report explains, some expansion is expected upon future update with further years of data, compounded by recent overcome rates by biologic age increasingly a factor in modern standard of care. However, comparing percentages at each of ages 68, 69, and 70, 1-year relative survival ranged from 95%-96%, an insignificant difference that is related more to the smaller numerators (and so more random variation) at the older ages than to meaningful difference in the age-specific survival rates.

Key findings by age group. Year of diagnosis is strongly correlated with 1- and 5-year observed survival - older age was related to a lower risk of death in the subsequent 1- and 5-year period. The age-adjusted bladder cancer survival trends reported in the main report are stable at roughly 72-73 percent of relative survival. A detailed examination of 1-year survival rates by age group found 95-96 percent 1-year relative survival at each of ages 68, 69, 70, 71, 72, 74, 79, 81, and 89.

## 6.2. Interpretation of Results

While untreated high-grade T1 cancer risk was significantly associated with worse malignant prognosis, as was having one or more symptoms (bioscall sig) was associated with increased malignancy-specific death. Race and portrayal impact for the 70-84 age group, removing mention of insignificant and may be considered. This could also limit discussion to effective invasive treatment type for patients, stating they the lower risk cite twice the result for cystectomy, specified pre-treatment truly immune stachahn-ris but is a forgotten or post-impressive NMSR comments. Further commenter dialing stop institutions for inv for chemoir.sa miceo sint was detected the later agar co-group it is recurrent characteristics, ag is detected in patients, which could all be discussed. Good work on weeding and sending it in. Our life tables are also still outstanding.

Each of our Cox proportional hazards models paints a different picture for each age group. For patients younger than 60, there was no significant variable to predict worse cancer-specific survival. This could indicate that the older patients were dying elsewhere from other non-bladder cancer conditions. However, for the 45 to 59-year-olds, the ones with a stated 2 or more than 3 symptoms were at a 62% higher but non-statistically significant risk of death from bladder cancer. For the 60 to 69-year-olds with two or more symptoms, they had CMS with a stage 1, lower risk tumor wouldn't have chemotherapy for IR and IC as survival, increased, but insignificantly, risk of death from cancer of 51%. Even for the 70 to 84-year-olds, there were differences within patients treated with the same treatment type. Those receiving chemotherapy IR and also IC instillations with three or more symptoms, more normally take the irregular so this could indicate health impacts rather than purely investigation-based changes, had a cancer-specific survival rate 114% higher but non-significant risk of death for cancer; possibly since these people were very ill.

# 7. Clinical Implications

# 7.1. Tailoring Treatment Based on Age

# 7.2. Supportive Care and Palliative Options

# 8. Future Directions

Innovation in bladder cancer is a publication from the European Association of Urology (EAU) where the changes and advances in bladder cancer are reported yearly. The adverse features of T1 disease are no longer stage or grade, an area where we need to focus. Intravesical treatments show good results in not only preventing the development of a muscle-invasive bladder cancer but producing a durable response. There is already work on the treatment of the elderly. We need to focus on how best to treat elderly patients should they progress to muscle-invasive bladder cancer. Management tools for prompt referral and the capacity of units to conduct timely oncological resections will also define improvements in care. Sathianan et al. 32 have shown that resection type for bladder cancer is not associated with the weekend effect in a retrospective series where worldwide reductions in emergency department visits have been reported.

Future directions. We found that survival disparities by age at diagnosis were consistent regardless of sample, country, tumor stage distribution, and study period. Ireland exhibits lower relative survival estimates, which was expected given the lower stage at diagnosis in the UK. The common observation of better age-specific survival for those younger patients diagnosed in recent years is relatively new and requires further verification from other countries. Perhaps it reflects an improvement in treatment against more aggressive tumors which disproportionately affect younger people. As the age profile is shifting towards an increasing percentage of older people, more and more people are living well with and surviving their bladder cancer diagnosis, and therefore, old age is no longer considered a risk factor for survival by government policy. The risk factors for time to cystectomy by age are also explored in Steevens et al.

## 8.1. Potential Areas for Further Research

The golden standard for calculating the stage and cell grade of a bladder cancer is from biopsies. Biopsies are subject to large discretionary variation throughout the United States. The stage and very importantly, the cell grade, if inferior by 2 stages classifies a bladder cancer as noninvasive or invasive. No information was available on muscle invasion at the time a bladder cancer was first diagnosed nor absolutely when the grade is known to the medic even if a good staging procedure were completed, 5 and 4-year survival rates as currently calculated do not provide evidence on health effects. Discovery of the disease at an earlier stage and the physician's interpretation of the statistically secondary evidence 5-year survival rate after 5 years, all provided more clinical evidence based for a wide range of ages, all ages with diagnosed and tissues excised range from the preteenager to centurion survival rates shown.

This study provided a first cut of the evidence related to whether age and stage at diagnosis were associated with the changes in age-specific bladder cancer survival rates observed (rates steady for ages 45-54, increasing rates for ages 55-64, and decreasing rates for ages 65-70 from 1994 through 2002). Extant provision cited here is by no means comprehensive but suggests a few areas for further research. Included among these might be stage and tumor cell grade due to their large associated changes in survival, already documented as systematic differences across age at bladder cancer diagnosis, and associated large changes in age-specific incidence of bladder cancer. Mortality (of all causes) due to competing risks including high and low staged cancer has been shown in the Surveillance, Epidemiology, and End Results (SEER) registries to more than account for the decreasing 5-year or 10-year relative survival rates reported here.

## 8.2. Innovations in Treatment and Care

Bladder cancer treatment has evolved little over the past 20 years. Since the 2000s, intravesical chemo- and immunotherapy trials have not shown significant survival benefit. However, behind absolute outcomes, there can be age-related differences. This last analysis also clearly shows that for certain age groups both the outcomes and benefit from adjuvant treatments are different. The optimal care best first be defined for the most vulnerable, before this 'enrichment' of the population in bladder cancer trials becomes standard care if results are extrapolated to fit all patients and not appreciating survivorship. Overall, the treatment landscape for both NMIBC and MIBC will change, for a multitude of reasons. In MIBC, radical treatment paradigms are changing and evolving. Moreover, innovative treatments and tools aim to individualise care for the population, considering specific age-related issues. It is expected that the above developments will have a positive impact on patient outcomes in the very near future.

In general, the provision of care for the aging population in Europe, and elsewhere, is influenced by changes in the demography and epidemiology of cancer. Remarkable advances in healthcare have led to an increase in life expectancy; the more years lived, the higher the risk of finally developing cancer. However, the more years a person lives, the less disease-free years are to be expected. Therefore, the European population is ever-aging, and with that comes an increasing cancer burden. The innovation in caring for an ever older cancer population becomes an urgent issue, because: (1) acceptable treatment delays in the general population may impose a too high burden on the aging cohort; and (2) adjuvant treatment should be critically revised, with a focus on multimorbidity and the individual survivorship of people with a wealth of diseases. Healthcare is currently facing an increased median age of the population, partly as 10-year survival for most cancers is increasing across Western societies.

# 9. Conclusion

# Bladder Cancer Survival Rates in Relation to Age: A Comprehensive Analysis

# 1. Introduction to Bladder Cancer

Broadly speaking, age impacts cancer survival: older patients demonstrate lower survival rates due to a combination of factors such as disease biology, health status, organ function, and complications from cancer therapies. The relationship between age and survival can be further delineated by cancer site. When we consider age as a factor affecting bladder cancer survival specifically, the findings are muddled. Predictors of survival mentioned earlier (especially the latter two, which encompass the concept of functional status) are problems often associated with the elderly. Conclusions with regard to bladder cancer survival and age from the broad cancer literature have not addressed the identified complexities outlined above. The decreased bladder cancer-specific survival seen in the elderly may primarily be the result of factors unique to age, or to the unrelated presence of comorbidities so often seen in the elderly. In this essay, we will specifically address predicted survival, and survival by treatment delivered, based on age alone.

As the cause of more than 19,000 annual deaths in the United States and with a worldwide share of 200,000 deaths per year, bladder cancer is considered a major global health issue. Non-muscle invasive bladder cancer (NMIBC) is the most prevalent variety, comprising 70-80% of all diagnosed cases. When treated early, the immediate outlook for patients with NMIBC is frequently promising. The other 20-30% of cases involve invasion of the detrusor muscle, and more often than not, cases are identified at a later point. These patients, classified as having muscle-invasive bladder cancer (MIBC), are at a much higher risk of poor prognosis and death.

In this paper, we will delve into the topic of bladder cancer survival rates. We aim to explore the realistic outlook for patients diagnosed with bladder cancer, based on the age of the patient. With this outline for our essay in mind, let's take a quick look into what is known about bladder cancer to get started.

## 1.1. Definition and Types of Bladder Cancer

Invasive bladder cancer can be further classified into two other categories. Urothelial carcinoma of the bladder affects almost all bladder cancer patients. Urothelial carcinomas can also be divided into two subgroups: gross or non-papillary and superficial or papillary bladder tumors. Papillary tumors do not grow flat and have finger-like fibers. The flat non-papillary variety is less common compared to the latter and is considered a type of bladder cancer. Squamous cell carcinomas and adenocarcinomas are further categories of invasive bladder cancer seen in bladder cancer patients. Squamous cell carcinomas attack the bladder lining cells undergoing metaplastic changes, which tend to resist transformation.

Bladder cancer, being referred to as a disease, can be explained as a growth of abnormal tissue in the bladder, replacing the natural cells. The probability of suffering from bladder cancer varies drastically based on factors such as sex, age, race, genetics, and lifestyle habits. Each bladder cancer case is different in terms of its cause, leading to the classification of various types based on progression and characteristics. The two main types are non-invasive bladder cancer, which does not spread through the muscle or invade other tissues, and invasive bladder cancer, which spreads through the muscle and invades the tissues.

## 1.2. Epidemiology and Prevalence

The disease is generally diagnosed after 65 years of age; the median age at diagnosis is 73 years, with the highest frequency at 79 years. The peak in diagnosis occurs between 70 and 74 years of age, which is the youngest group to be diagnosed with cancer, while the peak of death is reported among those aged 80 and over. The age-standard incidence is 22.3% in the age group older than 50 and 44 cases per 100,000 inhabitants in the age group between 70 and 79. Furthermore, it seems that there is an increasing incidence of bladder cancer. Among the many factors that contribute to this frequency is the percentage of elderly patients, given the increase in oncological diseases with advancing age. The prevalence of bladder carcinomas therefore also increases with age; given the increasing life expectancy, it is conceivable that there will also be an increase in the number of tumors, and consequently the number of invasive procedures.

Bladder cancer is the tenth most common cancer worldwide (8th in men and 17th in women), with 549,000 new cases and 200,000 deaths estimated in 2018. In 73% of cases, it is diagnosed at an early stage and the 5-year survival is greater than 70%, while for tumors diagnosed at a later stage, the 5-year survival is around 20%. Although located in the same anatomical site, bladder carcinomas can have different characteristics and behavior, so much so that it is defined as a complex and highly heterogeneous disease. We can begin to divide the bladder cancer in an oversimplifying way basing ourselves on the etiological agent: we can have bladder cancer associated with chemical agents such as tobacco, occupational exposure or after alkylating chemotherapy; we can also have non-chemical carcinomas, such as Schistosomes associated carcinomas, and carcinomas induced by radiation treatment for prostate cancer. Moreover, it is two times more common in non-Hispanic whites than in blacks and is rare in other racial groups. It affects mostly men, with a male-to-female ratio of 3:1 in non-Hispanic whites and 2:1 in blacks.

## 2. Factors Influencing Bladder Cancer Survival

Adjuvant treatment, as it is understood in other solid tumors, only has the potential to improve outcome in muscle-invasive bladder cancer if it diminishes the risk of distant metastases and requires an assessment of the risk of micrometastases far from the site of primary disease. Most patients with early stage, non-metastatic, transitional cell carcinoma of the bladder will never develop metastatic disease or die from it. Current international guidelines are focused on attempting to identify those patients that could be and would benefit from aggressive adjuvant treatment. Lymphovascular invasion and lymph node metastases are the most important prognostic factors both for survival in transitional cell carcinoma of the bladder and for selecting patients that might benefit from adjuvant chemotherapy. Age is also increasingly recognized as an important consideration when chemo-decision is made following radical cystectomy. Hematological and non-hematological toxicities of chemotherapy can be increased in elderly patients. Moreover, elderly patients are at increased risk of mortality from non-cancer competing causes. Hematological toxicity is the major reason elderly patients do not receive cisplatin-based combination chemotherapy. It has been shown that the risk of neutropenia increased with the age of the recipient, especially after 70 years. Furthermore, elderly patients receiving cisplatin-based neoadjuvant chemotherapy have higher grade 3/4 complications, such as digestive toxicity, hematological toxicity, infection, and fatigue. Chemotherapy itself, and its toxicities, partially contribute to the decreased adherence to oncological treatments in elderly people. Based on the increasing evidence of the real-life co-existing comorbidities in elderly patients undergoing cystectomy and the potential benefit of adjuvant systemic treatment, the future therapeutic management should endorse elderly people to also undergo this therapeutic option after radical cystectomy.

Survival in bladder cancer is determined by a variety of factors including patient and tumor characteristics, the effectiveness of local control measures, and the risk of distant metastases. The most consistent, well-established prognostic factors are pathological stage, histology, and lymphovascular invasion. Other host-related factors studied to date are either of modest independent importance or require validation in independent materials. Tumor-related factors usually impact on outcome through an effect on the risk of metastases. Changes that increase tumor size and invasiveness, as indicated by higher pathological stage, and the likelihood of metastases reduce survival. It is also clear that the physiological state of the patient, as measured by the glomerular filtration rate, is important in determining outcome. Elderly and infirm patients are likely to die with rather than from bladder cancer. In common with all solid tumors, comorbid medical conditions and frailty, which increase with chronological age, play an increasing part in determining the overall risk of death.

## 2.1. Age as a Significant Factor

Surprisingly, little information has been published regarding bladder cancer treatments and outcomes in older adults. In a systematic review of the literature over the period 1990 to 2000, we encountered only 11 publications that addressed issues such as the impact of radical cystectomy on survival, the use of intravesical therapy, or outcomes after systemic chemotherapy in patients older than 65 or older than 75 years of age. The disproportionately low number of investigators reporting on the care of older adults reflects widespread normalization of ageism in cancer care. Ageism reflects the bias that values the young over older adults and results in discriminatory clinical practices which, in turn, lead to lower access to life-sustaining treatments and hence lower survival rates. The goal of the present study was to determine the role of age as a factor influencing overall survival in a group of Polish patients diagnosed with primary bladder cancer for whom solid and reliable follow-up was available.

Survival rates for superficial and invasive bladder cancer patients vary considerably. Many clinical and pathological factors have been shown to affect survival in cancer patients. Among these, the patient's age at the time of diagnosis plays a substantial role in the prognosis of many malignant diseases. Older patients have a greater risk of death due to many diseases, including cancer. Comparatively little is known about the effect of histological subtype and grade, as well as the stage of the disease at the time of diagnosis, on the overall survival of the patients from a defined study population where computational statistics and appropriate visualization methods were used.

## 2.2. Other Contributing Factors

As a result, while age is a well-documented contributory factor that can affect cancer outcomes, this does not mean that cancer in the elderly is essentially hopeless. The thorough influence of age on bladder cancer mortality and discussion of the subject are subjects on which there has been little emphasis. This is of concern since drug discovery and initial clinical studies continue to be concentrated almost entirely on younger cancer patients, directly giving the drug not only the allowance of sole use of drugs to younger people but also examining them in an older setting that is more pragmatic.

Factors beyond age that contribute to survival rates, such as sex, race, insurance, and tumor characteristics, are believed to play roles in these disparities. Other variables, like comorbid health conditions, stage at diagnosis, and type of treatments, are also well established to affect the prognosis of the disease. Some of these issues can be more influenced by patient age; for instance, patients in their 70s are more likely not to receive standard of care treatments following surgery, which can weaken their prognosis. On the other hand, age of a patient can possibly have no influence on some of these other measures. Instead, as a proxy for comorbid conditions or physiological age, this influence could be explained by apparent survival data, which can describe how much more or less likely a patient is to die of cancer in comparison with a similar person of the same education, sex, race, and income going through society.

# 3. Data Sources and Methodology

Data have been provided for both comparative and selective data quality for the first consultation with the clinician and to include all patients irrespective of the previously treated stage of the disease. More detailed information on data selection is available from an online manual that provides detailed and comprehensive documentation. This manual has been created to demonstrate data collection details and provides a transcript of every cancer found, with the time this cancer was first diagnosed, the unique patient registration number, and additional data that is relevant for building survival models. Data collection is beneficial when only 1 case is registered in a country for rare types of tumor, then only one entry will be attributed. National survival is also provided for all of our cases. Data collection, surpassing, taxonomy, and definitions are provided from an internationally accepted source. When no data is available or partial occurrences are present, the entries are not listed.

This study utilizes SURVCAT, which is a product of the HealthData of Global Health Data Exchange. The electronic database provides population-based, individual-level survival data on patients diagnosed with cancer, including bladder cancer. It contains survival data for 39 countries and relies on a large amount of incidence data derived from cancer registries, especially those in younger established registries. The dataset is designed to be representative of all countries and regions in terms of human development level, income level, world region, and patient anonymity coverage. The registry of this data follows ethical rules, and the IRB of VU Medical Center Council is responsible for assuring the study is conducted following ethical standards. The data includes over 100,000 individuals diagnosed with bladder cancer. It is built from 105 registries which are systematically reviewed to maintain the dataset.

## 3.1. Population-Based Studies

Supplementary filed Tables S12, S18, S19, S22, S23 showed the result of ASR of Relative 5-Year Survival Rates of BC by Age Group and Registries from around the world, including the USA. The estimate of the Americas registry would be needed in a multi-country model to accurately estimate the age effects beyond the USA or the comparison country. The SEER monographs and some publications are the only source where the estimates needed for a complete appraisal of how disease progression affects the disease among the comparison countries and registries. However, a random effects model with only the USA data needs sufficient data only from the comparison country to identify the additional time period parameter for each grouping of ages as in the Surveillance, Epidemiology, and End Results (SEER). The results emphasize the data dependencies, especially for measures of older age and for comparing registries not in the SEER program. The ASR dropped to 14.3 among ages 80-84, indicating a steep survival decline and small population size. In the oldest age group (85+) in the presence of bladder cancer, less than 0.1% of the US population per year receives treatment (936 individuals in 2014) (assuming 5-year prevalence = incidence for the oldest age group of approximately 70-100 per 100,000/yr). The analytic age that separated only from 0, which would have been impossible to bond with the prior small population, dropping down to 5 years of age. It was left in the oldest age strata that we stratification just as a categorization of new cases diagnosed and older ages cases as an intermediate computation. The survival rate and the associated magnitude of the APe, calculated here as age prevalence of stage. Stage is truncated the survival differences and was selected to capture early disease. Because of population size constraints (e.g., limited cases appearing or surviving beyond 5 years after diagnosis), for this reason, 5-year relative survival information was chosen to validate the funnel plot statistical model.

At the population level, different research agencies within countries have been conducting their own large epidemiologic studies in an ongoing effort to provide and interpret a comprehensive profile for the disease processes and describe survival rates for various demographic categories, including age groups as discussed in the Introduction section. Here, we compiled and explored the difference in 5-year relative survival rates of the USA and other European countries, including the UK, Estonia, Denmark, Israel, Spain, and Slovenia (Fig. 3), and Slovenia. Countries with their estimates included with age 0+ are Denmark and the US (Surveillance, Epidemiology, and End Results: SEER-18 and SEER-9), but it was not possible to learn about the mode of age classification based on the open data from the reference. Yet, concerning the remaining countries, that is, the UK, Estonia, Israel, Spain, and Slovenia, a difference in 5-year relative net survival rates based on age group information was presented. For example, the UK (OS) displayed the observed proportion of women alive based on age group at diagnosis. A portion of this "proportion alive" measure is then averaged over 5 years and converted to "net survival" through an algorithm. General information about the supervised models showed that the NB-REG-tool was employed by the US, and the Pohar-Perme model is employed based on the UK (E&W), Spain (south), and Slovenia. The reference states that Segi-Doll is a tool based on direct adjustment and listed-based coverage from East, South Switzerland (Switz), and Macedonia. It not only provides a 5-year relative net percentage of the people alive by each 5-year interval but they have also performed direct age adjustment.

## 3.2. Survival Rate Calculation Methods

Despite evidence to suggest that younger patients of working age with muscle-invasive and non-muscle-invasive bladder cancer manifest slightly different clinical and pathological features to their older counterparts, there is little consensus as to the outcome measures that should be used when assessing outcomes in age-defined populations. However, for a reader to take heed of the results and draw changes from this paper, it is essential to understand that older women with muscle-invasive and non-muscle-invasive bladder cancer are often excluded from clinical trials for treatment. Even if older women are included in trials, their findings in a mixed age and mixed sex "bladder cancer" group can at times be challenging to extrapolate to stand-alone data sets due to potentially confounding variables. As previously mentioned, bladder cancer in younger men and women has not shown to be significantly different. Furthermore, little has been published specifically in relation to male NMIBC patients.

It is unclear how different authors performed the survival rate calculations for different age groups, but consider the use of Mantel-Cox (log-rank) tests and Kaplan-Meier curves to determine patient subgroup competitiveness and overall survival in the context of "competing risk" due to death from other causes. It is possible that authors have not performed subgroup-complementary statistical tests in their original investigations to support survival rate estimations, and therefore, original studies of all age groups below 90 have been included in this review. There is no widely agreed upper age limit at which to operate on those older patients presenting with muscle-invasive and non-muscle-invasive bladder cancer, and patients are treated according to disease status, co-morbidities, and general life expectancy, helping to inform the best treatment regime to follow.

# 4. Bladder Cancer Survival Rates Across Different Age Groups

# 4.1. Pediatric and Young Adult Populations

## 4.2. Adult Populations

# 4.3. Geriatric Populations

# 5. Trends and Patterns in Bladder Cancer Survival Rates

In order to provide a comprehensive view of bladder cancer survival rates in relation to age, we also analyze the time trends by socioeconomic region of residence. Age was available in four categories. "Trends" refer to changes in survival rates over a sufficient period of time. "Patterns" refer to the levels at which particular survival rates may be observed. In such countries, more healthcare resources can be dedicated to this cohort of population; more incipient and, therefore, easily managed cases are seen, in which a cure is likely to be more feasible. These little differences also have an effect on survival. To better substantiate these statements, we provide a comprehensive analysis of bladder cancer survival rates in relation to age, by socioeconomic region of residence.

Historical changes in survival rates unveiled some important patterns. For instance, there was a clear increase from 1975 to 1979 up to 1980-1984 that may be at least partially explained by the rise in bladder cancer incidence. The 5-year relative survival was 81% in Europe between 1978 and 1992, similar to what was to be expected between 1985 and 1989 and 1997-2002. Or, in other words, no great changes had been produced by the introduction of new potentially effective complementary treatments, in the control of costs, in the availability of these modalities or in the general support to the management of elderly population with advanced disease.

Also, the description of trends and patterns is valuable in the comprehensive evaluation of survival rate outcomes, but when making age-comparisons, the analysis of survival data is expected to play a quite secondary role.

## 5.1. Historical Changes

In the literature, we found comparable results at different ranges of age and analysis span. Regarding OS, a significant change could have happened between mid-2000s and 2010s: Herr found that men aged more than 75 between 2002 and 2013 showed an increment in OS compared to the previous cohort. These results suggest a major contribution due to treatments rather than OS, considering that during the same period an increase in non-invasive cancers occurred. This is in line with our results and increases confidence in historical adjustments; in this sense, many aspects must be considered such as potential data variations, differences in the survival rate analyses, or the coincidence of some of our earlier studies within the updated analyses period, mainly including the ones on NMIBC patients.

Historical trends of bladder cancer survival could provide a better understanding of the temporal dynamics associated with the oncological outcomes after the implementation of new therapeutic strategies. In our analysis, chronologically ordered cohorts have been classified into age quartiles in order to perform a comprehensive investigation on trends and findings from both recent and previous literature. Previous studies were performed in different ages and dates from 1992 to 2009; survival rates were variously classified either by age, in terms of composite analyses, or focusing on one specific treatment. We observed that the women-only quartile of those aged 79–94 between 2008 and 2017 showed a slight decrease in OS, while the 4-year

CSS was higher compared to the previous three quartiles (78.8% vs. 29.3, 38.3, and 55.1%, respectively). Conversely, the CG SCC females over the age of 79 classified as the 5th quintile between 1973 and 2012 displayed an increase in CSS.

## 5.2. Regional Disparities

However, during the eighties, there was an important increase in survival for the 75–84-year-old population (data not shown), with higher mortality rates back into the nineties and early 2000s. The new more recent cancer therapeutics could be, thus, one of the reasons for the reversal of this trend. We thus went on to test these two groups amongst the population aged 85 and above. This idea is even confirmed by the trends identified in Figure 20 of the greater increase in the OS over CSS in this last cohort. Figure 24 represents the geographical disparities in survival ratios between OS and CSS of bladder cancer patients aged 85+. It is much easier shown that patients from the Midwest have a much higher - and keeping increasing - trend in the OS/CSS ratio (e.g., 2015 is 4 ± 1.1) compared to all of the other regions (the closest being the South with the 2015 OS/CSS ratio is 2.8 ± 1.05).

No significant regional disparities in age-specific overall survival (OS) were identified for patients aged 50–64 and 65–74. The 75–84 group had lower OS in males from the Midwest and the West than in the South. Similarly, females aged 75–84 showed lower OS in the Midwest and the West compared to the South. Patients aged 85+ had lower OS in the West compared to the other regions in both genders. No significant regional disparities in cancer-specific survival (CSS) were identified for the 50–64, 65–74, and 75–84 age groups.

5.2. Regional Disparities

# 6. Challenges and Limitations in Survival Rate Studies

The Netherlands Cancer Registry, which includes all patients diagnosed with cancer or with a progressive tumor at death, indicates patterns and trends and could potentially inform outcomes even in the absence of follow-up. In many countries, there is no clear definition of dependence. In addition, "frequently" means a wide range of values from 2.5 to 90. Also, these authors did not consider the problem of dependence in their analysis. One last necessary consideration is the role of primary versus recurrent tumors in the calculation of 5-year net survival rates. For clinical trial results, one can imagine that all primary tumors are included. In a registry, this is quite different, at least in North America. Only 58% of the tumors entered into two large urological registry databases were primary. It is not clear whether such a distribution is reflected in general populations.

The current study had some limitations and challenges that may need to be discussed. However, the publication length limit did not permit us to address these challenges in detail. This section provides comprehensive insights into these limitations. For instance, there was no consensus on the number of cases and the length of the study follow-up. The lowest recommended number of bladder cancer cases was 50. Some authors recommended follow-up periods of 5 years, whereas others considered that 3 years were acceptable.

## 6.1. Data Accuracy and Completeness

Data not accurately recorded or not appearing in the medical record, particularly as they relate to diagnosis and comorbidity, could introduce biases in the reported analyses. Confounding factors exist that may not be completely controlled for across the studies or data sources. The SEER registry is designed to be representative of the US population. However, MCC may be under-represented as they are more likely to be diagnosed with bladder cancer in the community setting, particularly at older ages. MCC are also less likely to receive definitive treatment for their cancer, so those patients that are included may be a biased, healthier population. Larger databases are available but the comorbidity information is limited and not as dynamic. Data derived from electronic medical records or have been an effort of targeted data collection, including data collections processes that are part of the norm as the patients progress on the standard care process, are less susceptible to bias.

Results will only be as good as the data collected, and in many populations, data collected for those patients with bladder cancer may not be adequate. Resulting analysis, for example, from SEER may omit data on nodal status if these surgical specimens are not routinely processed. An inadequate proportion of survival estimates were reported in an adjusted manner. In addition, only a few data sources capture comorbidity information.

## 6.2. Confounding Variables

Given these results, and supported by the established propensity of cancer to develop after a long period of inflammation, we now test the hypothesis that tumor markers, in particular Carcinoembryonic Antigen (CEA) and Carbohydrate Antigen 19-9 (CA19-9), are also independently associated with other malignancies in PSC patients. A significant number of PSC-CC patients have raised tumor markers prior to CCA diagnosis. For the remaining patients, 25% have at least one raised tumor marker, a finding not entirely dissimilar to population background (revised here, for comparison with later findings). A logical explanation for the part of all patients with raised tumor marker and subsequently diagnosed with CCA is as "early CCA", such as the reported "incidental gallbladders" where histopathological examination reveals CCA which was asymptomatic or just presents as cholecystitis (elevation of CA 19-9) [5].

As with many observational data studies, there are a number of confounding variables that may influence the interpretation of overall and age sub-stratified cancer-specific and all-cause survival rates. There are a large number of variables that should correspond either directly or, more commonly, indirectly, to patient health and hence impact survival rates. This includes the common cancer data confounders such as cancer tumor grade and stage. To attempt to control for these, we have intensively reviewed the literature, incorporating new evidence from the population-based Singapore Cancer Registry, to produce comprehensive grade and stage-specific cancer-specific survival curves for use in future meta-analyses and cancer policy. The values given are of direct clinical use, as they represent up-to-date OS curves stratified simultaneously by cancer stage and primary sclerosing cholangitis (PSC) status. We were able to identify evidence of cancerous invasion in 111 out of 151 patients (74.5%).

# 7. Clinical Implications and Recommendations

To optimize BCa care in consideration of the different age groups, the following possible recommendations could be made: Individualized treatment for pediatric-adolescent population: due to the rarity of the disease in this age group, pediatric-adolescent patients should be referred to experienced oncological centers. Rapid assessment by an expert multidisciplinary team and treatment in a high-volume center should be offered to adult patients. Primary surgery is recommended for the treatment of MIBC, particularly in the elderly who present a higher chance of complications and a generally poor tolerance to systemic therapy. For elderly not eligible for RADICALS but with a preserved ECOG-PS, treatment decision should be based on CGA. The decision to administer palliative chemotherapy in elderly patients should also be considered. The high level of comorbidity in elderly BC patients plays a key role in the quality of life of these patients, impacting on survival outcomes. The judicious use of the available novelties should occur by constantly sharing information and expectations with the patient, considering the benefits and risks of such treatments. Overall, optimal care should be an integrated personalized therapy for the single patient. Early detection through the establishment of massive screening programs oriented to high-risk population and the research of biomarkers can significantly increase the percentage of radical surgical resections. Plasma DNA might represent a novel predictive non-invasive tool for the modification of surveillance strategies after a diagnosis of BC. Implementation of geriatric assessment: Cancers are diseases typically occurring in people aged 65 years and older. As this growing population lives longer, the risk of developing new cancers while receiving care for an earlier cancer is an area of increasing importance. In this respect, bladder cancer in older people, with multiple comorbidities, malnutrition, have a functional dependency and psychosocial issues, impairs the functional capacity that affects the tolerance and pharmacokinetics of cancer therapies like chemotherapy. Some researchers argue that poor outcomes in certain cancer are associated with more acute physiologic changes. Conducting geriatric assessments in older patients can help identify priority problems and be leveraged to tailor more aggressive treatment systems specifically designed to address physical functioning. Doing a geriatric assessment will show how many older adults are potentially becoming victims to detrimental outcomes as a result of receiving more aggressive therapies. For these reasons, a geriatric assessment is recommended for those 70 years old and older.

Based on our comprehensive analysis of the impact of patient age on bladder cancer survival, some important recommendations can be made. Elderly patients present an impairment in their survival time for both nonmetastatic, MIBC, and mBC. Older patients included in clinical trials can represent a selected population with a better performance status impacting positively on the results of the trials. The eligibility criteria for clinical trials in bladder cancer do not usually consider comorbidities, geriatric syndromes, or a geriatric assessment that can help in the decision-making. On the basis of the current evidence on the biological behavior of this neoplasm, the quality of state-of-the-art urological and innovative patient multimodal treatment should not be conditioned by patient age. Different therapeutic strategies should be considered with a tailor-made approach according to the specific characteristics of each age class. Each treatment should be discussed at an experienced, multidisciplinary decision-making level, involving the patients and their caregivers.

## 7.1. Tailored Treatment Approaches by Age Group

In this regard, preliminary data suggest the independent prognostic role of age in this disease, particularly when treated with immunotherapy: it would be of interest to pool the patients enrolled in phase 2 and 3 with atezolizumab (IMvigor) in order to better weigh the impact of age on the prognosis of this population. Furthermore, developing specific randomized clinical trials could represent an effective tool to depict the attitudinal differences between age groups in undergoing conventional treatments such as radical cystectomy or immunotherapy. This approach, together with the unmet results from retrospective analysis, could help investigators to ameliorate the recruitment phase of the randomized clinical trials or the treatment in an everyday clinical setting of this peculiar population.

In line with the epidemiological data, we would like to outline some considerations, recommendations, and tailored treatment approaches in bladder cancer patients at different cut-off points by age groups, namely 40 to 49, 50 to 59, 60 to 69, 70 to 79, and 80 years. The rationale for such an approach lies behind the possibility to offer more personalized and specific management strategies, covering from diagnosis to disease monitoring, radiological and instrumental workflow (including conventional cystoscopy – namely "Cold Cup" as per commonly definition – or Narrow Band Imaging (NBI) cystoscopy), systemic treatments, comparative clinical trials as well as surgical options. In each section, we will further divide these patients in case of urothelial and non-urothelial bladder cancer. Furthermore, we will also provide the age group-independent general recommendations.

## 7.2. Importance of Early Detection and Intervention

An understanding of early-onset BC is crucial for public health and disease management. A recent study demonstrated that early diagnosis of BC, muscle-invasive BC in particular, would increase the survival rates. MIBC in young patients with early cancer detection is associated with a low risk of progression and favorable outcomes. In addition, the timely initiation of cancer treatment improves survival outcomes. Bladder-preserving therapy together with transurethral resection or partial cystectomy could be alternative BC treatment for early-onset patients, while muscle-invasive patients with worse pathologic responses undergoing radical cystectomy yield the best fit model. These findings may serve as arguments for healthcare instruments and policies. Therefore, our recommendation for clinicians is to start interventions as soon as possible to trigger and boost the immune system in early-onset patients.

Early detection and intervention are crucial for improving the survival rates of bladder cancer patients. Various retrospective studies showed that the 5-year overall survival, disease-specific survival, and progression-free survival of patients diagnosed with NMIBC were significantly better in patients with early-stage tumors and no carcinoma in situ. A recent population-based study involving early-onset patients with UTUC revealed that survival rates increased with earlier detection, thus demonstrating that UTUCs detected late were associated with poor survival outcomes. Furthermore, this study highlighted the positive impact of early detection, as patients with early-stage tumors showed significant improvements in their 5-year survival rates. Based on the results of our study, we similarly recommend that early-onset patients should undergo repeated screening for the early detection of BC, similar to early-onset UTUC patients.

# 8. Conclusion and Future Directions

There were no specific age groups at a greater risk, but survival rates remained reasonably similar until the age of 70, after which time a gradual decrease in survival was observed with increasing age. Clinically, these findings could serve as a useful tool, empowering general practitioners or healthcare professionals with less experience in the field of urology, to quantify the risk of death from bladder cancer for their elderly patients. Additional research could be performed to confirm these findings, as well as looking into the potential use of balancing risks and benefits of chemotherapy for elderly bladder cancer patients. Following on from the results of this study, a well-conducted and prospective multi-center trial, looking at the benefits of adjuvant chemotherapy for elderly patients with muscle-invasive bladder cancer, could be considered. Also, highlighting the lack of age-specific data on urothelial cancer (most studies combining all bladder and upper tract urothelium), future guidance should highlight the relevance of this data to help urological surgeons and oncologists in balancing the risks and benefits of intervention and conservative management of this disease. Moreover, randomized control trials have predominantly used chronological age as a criterion for patient selection, this study suggests that chronological age alone could be insufficient, diseases affect older people differently, such that age-stratified trials may improve our understanding of benefits and risks in this population. The potential clinical utility of these findings could have implications on how healthcare resources are used in treating elderly patients. Age-specific costs would, therefore, be a useful adjunct to clinical age-specific survival data. Also, highlighting the lack of age-specific data on urothelial cancer, future guidance should highlight the relevance of this data to help urological surgeons and oncologists in balancing the risks and benefits of intervention and conservative management of this disease.

Through the lens of seven main themes, this dissertation has comprehensively and methodically examined the relationship between age and bladder cancer survival rates. These various domains were thought to be relevant to the analysis of kidney cancer survival: the need to address multiple comparisons, age at diagnosis is dynamic, clinical course, the use of competing risks model, competing risk, test of heterogeneity in relative excess risk (i.e. as a test of trend), and the validity of using period approach to study cancer survival in general. By using the model of clinical course to understand the survival patterns, bladder cancer generally behaves more like neoplasms with a poor prognosis, such as stomach, liver, lung, pancreatic, and esophagus. This suggests that bladder cancer tends to kill its patients.

1. The prognosis for older bladder cancer patients is generally poor, with decreasing likelihoods of survival as the age at diagnosis progresses. The risk of death can be relatively high for such aging patients, exacerbated by the likelihood of recurrence or progression commonly related to the cancer type. Furthermore, higher age is a factor recognized to lower disease-specific survival rates and may be related to lesser chances of undergoing appropriate treatments. In fact, some imaging and cytological tests are not even recommended for the older population due to their ineffectiveness when used. Well, this holds as long as patients have no life-limiting comorbidities. Some studies even considered resection biopsies as candidates for observation even in cases of high-grade T1 disease among individuals with non-muscle-invasive urothelial cancer of the bladder. However, as has been discussed, those who are diagnosed with cancer at a younger age can seek treatments that are much more convenient due to their stronger and more robust overall health.

In developing and merging different sections on bladder cancer survival rates considering the age factor, several insights into how different age groups experience survival outcomes were discovered. Below is a summary of those key findings.

## 8.2. Potential Areas for Further Research

8.2.1. Tumor Biology and Variance in Response to Treatment Much has been written in the oncological literature about how "elderly physiology" is distinct from younger patients and it is postulated that these differences are the drivers for the age-related variation seen in oncological outcomes. One element of this is the concept of tumor biology – i.e., the intrinsic biological behavior of a malignancy. Strong evidence supports the concept that, say, an 80-year-old with muscle-invasive urothelial carcinoma has distinctly different tumor characteristics to, say, a 50-year-old with the same diagnosis. The older patient does worse because their tumor pathology or biology is less treatable (i.e., is more aggressive, responds to treatment less effectively, etc.).

As described in Chapter 7, there is an established association between increasing age and poorer survival following a diagnosis of muscle-invasive bladder cancer. The meta-regression model identified that overall survival at one year decreased by 4.5% for every additional 10 years in age. However, a deep understanding of why older patients with bladder cancer experience poorer outcomes has yet to be developed. There are several distinct areas of further research that may provide the detail which is lacking in this regard and ways in which this research can be conducted are also provided here.